MINDFULNESS
FOR CARERS

of related interest

Mindfulness-Based Interventions for Older Adults
Evidence for Practice
Carla Martins
ISBN 978 1 84905 487 4
eISBN 978 0 85700 880 0

Dementia – Support for Family and Friends
David Pulsford and Rachel Thompson
ISBN 978 1 84905 243 6
eISBN 978 0 85700 504 5

Mindful Therapeutic Care for Children
A Guide to Reflective Practice
Joanna North
ISBN 978 1 84905 446 1
eISBN 978 0 85700 840 4

Mindful Living with Asperger's Syndrome
**Everyday Mindfulness Practices to
Help You Tune in to the Present Moment**
Chris Mitchell
ISBN 978 1 84905 434 8
eISBN 970 0 85700 867 1

Mindfulness
FOR Carers

HOW TO MANAGE THE DEMANDS
OF CAREGIVING WHILE FINDING
A PLACE FOR YOURSELF

Dr Cheryl Rezek

Jessica Kingsley *Publishers*
London and Philadelphia

First published in 2015
by Jessica Kingsley Publishers
73 Collier Street
London N1 9BE, UK
and
400 Market Street, Suite 400
Philadelphia, PA 19106, USA

www.jkp.com

Library of Congress Cataloging in Publication Data
A CIP catalog record for this book is available from
the Library of Congress

British Library Cataloguing in Publication Data
A CIP catalogue record for this book is available
from the British Library

ISBN 978 1 84905 654 0
eISBN 978 1 78450 147 1

Printed and bound in Great Britain

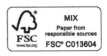

With grateful thanks to Tom Davey
for his assistance with this project.

CONTENTS

A NOTE ABOUT THE TEXT

To access the audio downloads that accompany this book go to: www.lifehappens-mindfulness.com/carers-audio/.

The terms carer and caregiver are used interchangeably throughout this book as they both refer to someone who is in the role of taking care of another person in a professional, parental, familial or friendship role.

Disclaimer: This book makes no claim to act as a cure or treatment of any conditions, nor does it advocate discontinuation of any intervention or treatment.

Do not listen to the audio material whilst driving or operating any machinery or item.

Take care of yourself:
You are your responsibility.

Introduction

Life happens

Life happens to each and every one of us. As much as we can take pleasure in the ups, part of the deal seems to be that there are downs too. Some aspects of our lives we can control and others we cannot. However, we always have the capacity within ourselves to choose our outlook on life, despite it feeling like a struggle to maintain a positive attitude at times.

Carergivers are often a group in society who are particularly vulnerable to feeling stressed, worried and frustrated about life. The vast range of demands that come with caregiving, whether it be physical, psychological or social can sometimes feel like a great strain to carry. The mindfulness approach can be of excellent value to people who are stressed and who are looking for something to help them develop greater inner stability, resilience and more management of their thoughts and emotions. Added to this, it not only has the important benefit of helping to reduce stress but it can also assist with reducing anxiety and depression.

What does this book offer you?

This book offers an introduction to mindfulness and how it can be applied to assisting carers manage their situations and experiences. A brief history of mindfulness and its key concepts will be summarised, followed by an outline of how mindfulness can be used for carers and the research on it.

There are numerous short practices within the text, which can be tried out at intervals as you are reading through it. A step-by-step guide is included to show you how to go about the practices that are available on the MP3 download (audio track), go to www.lifehappens-mindfulness.com/carers-audio/ when you see this symbol: ◀). You'll notice that it is very straightforward with no attempts to put you into an altered state.

It is advised that you try all the practices in the book as well as those from the MP3 download at least once. You can then begin to choose the practices you feel work best for you and take part in them on a regular enough basis for them to have an impact on your life. It is important to make time for yourself every day, or at least every few days, to carry out a practice. This will, when combined with the approach, provide you with a base that can continue its positive impact long-term. Remember the more you do it the greater the benefits.

Part 1

MINDFULNESS –
WHAT IS IT AND HOW CAN
IT BE OF USE TO ME?

CHAPTER 1

The Hustle and Bustle of Life

As the majority of us have felt at some point, life can feel like it's going a 100 miles an hour and we struggle to keep up. This book will give you ideas on how you can find some calm amongst what can at times feel like mayhem. Through reading the different sections, doing the practices and listening to the audio tracks ◀», you will find that you can begin to acquire a clearer perspective on your life. It will provide you with a foundation that can be a source of balance and steadiness in it, enabling you to give yourself more choice to live your life with a greater sense of control.

For carers, it can be difficult to maintain a balanced wellbeing and easy to feel tired from demanding responsibilities. In turn, these feelings can escalate into low self-esteem, depression, anxiety or a general level of distress and exhaustion that can come about over time. The ideas in this book will encourage you to consider your current situation and help you to understand what in your life, both past and present, has influenced how you currently think, feel and react.

If you have chosen to read this, it is possible that you are: (a) a carer or caregiver and (b) experiencing some kind of distress. However, mindfulness can be useful in helping to appreciate the good experiences we have too, which can so frequently be overshadowed. With the consistent use of the practices, there will be times in the day that you can attend to something good, rather than neglecting the present and fretting over what happened earlier or what other tasks you have to do later. Here is an introductory practice to start you off so you can get an idea of what is going on in your mind in the present moment.

Mindfulness practice: A moment of stillness

This practice is a simple but effective way to begin to understand what mindfulness is about.

Sit in stillness for two minutes, whilst paying attention to what is going through your mind.

- Were there any sensations? Did anything pop into your mind? Perhaps thoughts relating to your caregiving duties came to mind. If so, were they good or difficult thoughts?

- Did you feel calmer or more stressed? Why do you think that was? Note down as many thoughts and sensations as you can remember. When we take the time to sit in stillness, often our minds can be overrun by all the things queuing for our attention.

• In the following sections, the mindfulness practices can help to develop your focused attention, allowing you to take a step back from all of these thoughts and feelings.

SUMMARY

• Carers are particularly susceptible to stress due to their demanding responsibilities.

• Mindfulness can help you to appreciate the good experiences of your life more often.

CHAPTER 2

What is Mindfulness?

What is mindfulness?

Mindfulness is about bringing your attention to:

- what is happening within you and around you
- in this moment.

(Rezek 2012)

It is the process of paying attention to yourself – to your feelings, thoughts, actions, and choices – all within the context of now. It requires curiosity to find out what is going on in your mind and body. By focusing attention on yourself, you can raise your awareness of what you think and feel, and learn a different way of managing them.

Generally, carers can be worriers, as it often comes with the role. Carers' minds are usually filled with thoughts of how they can best support the person or people they care for, but frequently carers ignore their own needs. The stresses imposed on us in day-to-day life can so often be pushed into the corners of our minds.

However, they will always find a way out of the shadows and show themselves in other ways which can sometimes be damaging, such as in the form of physical or mental health problems. A mindful approach to life permits us to bring these stresses into the light so that we can deal with them in helpful ways.

Whistle-stop tour on the history of mindfulness

Mindfulness has stretched across more than 2500 years, being an element of Buddhist philosophies (Allen, Chambers and Knight 2006). Central features of Buddhist practices are meditations where the focal point is on breathing techniques encouraging us to be present in the moment and directing kindness towards ourselves and others. These practices have made their way over to Western societies in the last 30 or 40 years. In 1979, colleagues at the University of Massachusetts Medical Center, Boston, USA, developed a programme incorporating these mindfulness meditation practices for people who were in physical distress. This programme was labelled Mindfulness-Based Stress Reduction (MBSR) (McBee 2003).

Meditation? That's not for me...

It is not uncommon for the term meditation to raise a few eyebrows. Sometimes in society, it is seen as a trancelike state. This is most definitely not the case in the context of mindfulness where rather than shutting off, it promotes sharpening your attention on the here and now. It helps you to be open to your present thoughts in a more complete and non-reactive way (Rezek 2012).

Mindfulness practice: Let's go for a walk

Focusing your attention on your automatic functions can ground you, and this walking practice can help to settle you when stress is troubling you. Try it when you can feel your frustrations growing.

- Take a walk wherever is convenient. Keeping your eyes half closed, bring your attention to the sensations of walking. Now slow down your pace. Feel the changes in pressure as you place your feet on the ground, the rhythm of your footsteps and the motion of your arms.

- Acknowledge any emotions that come to mind. Take a mental step back from such an active involvement in the environment. Keep your focus on your body and the sensation of moving slowly and with attention. Continue to observe your breathing as a space forms between you and the outside world.

- Take a moment to appreciate this moment, knowing you can carry this sense of quietness and clarity with you when you move back into your everyday activities.

SUMMARY

- Mindfulness is the process of paying attention to yourself in the context of now.

- It's embedded in Buddhist philosophies dating back 2500 years.

CHAPTER 3

Proof that Mindfulness Helps

In the last decade, research on mindfulness has increased markedly with its effects on a number of issues having been investigated. Carers fall into various groups depending on their situations. For example, you may be a carer of an elderly parent or sick child or work as a formal carer in your job. The following list shows some of the evidence for the use of mindfulness for various groups of carers.

Mindfulness for people employed as formal care workers

- A mindfulness-based programme lowered distress by 35 per cent amongst health workers; the positive effects remained three months later (Martín-Asuero and García-Banda 2010).

- Mindfulness can assist social workers in having a positive wellbeing, develop their sense of identity and awareness of the self and maintain a work–life balance (Shier and Graham 2010).

- Mindfulness increased resilience and general health, and decreased stress in nurses and midwives (Foueur *et al.* 2013).

- Mindfulness had a significant effect on the health and wellbeing of nurses employed in a corporate setting (Bazarko *et al.* 2013) and on nurses and nurse aides' life satisfaction, burnout symptoms and relaxation (MacKenzie, Poulin and Seidman-Carlson 2006).

- A mindfulness programme assisted nursing home staff by reducing their stress-related psychological distress (McBee 2003).

- Mindfulness decreases burnout, emotional exhaustion and compassion fatigue and increases empathy and compassion in healthcare professionals including physicians, nurses, social workers, physical therapists and psychologists (Shapiro *et al.* 2005; Goodman and Schorling 2012).

- Mindfulness increased levels of self-reported empathy in medical and premedical students (Shapiro, Schwartz and Bonner 1998) and reduced burnout, depression, anxiety and stress in primary care physicians (Fourtney *et al.* 2013).

- Mindfulness was one intervention that helped reduce the consequences of stress in physicians (Regehr, Glancy and Leblanc 2014).

- In palliative care settings, mindfulness training decreased burnout and moral distress (Rushton, Kaszniak and Halifax 2013).

- Mindfulness-based mentoring increased team functioning and 'teamness' amongst staff at an inpatient psychiatric hospital; these effects remained one year later (Singh *et al.* 2006a).

Mindfulness for parents or carers of children

- Mindful parenting can reduce parental stress and resulting parental reactivity, stop the transfer of unhelpful parenting habits to future generations and improve marital functioning and co-parenting (Bögels, Lehtonen and Restifo 2010).

- A mindfulness programme had a positive effect on parents of children with special educational needs or chronic conditions, reducing the stress symptoms of the parents by over 30 per cent and reducing their troubled mood by almost 60 per cent (Minor *et al.* 2006).

- Training in the practice of mindfulness helped parents of children with autism reduce stress, increase satisfaction in their parenting skills and increase their child's social skills with more social interaction (Singh *et al.* 2007).

- Mindfulness helped foster parents with stress around some aspects of parenting (Baker 2014).

- Mindfulness training for parents and educators of children with special needs led to significant reductions in stress and anxiety and increased mindfulness, self-compassion and personal growth even after two months (Benn *et al.* 2012).

- Parents and educators of children with special needs also showed a significant positive change in their feeling competent in their relating abilities after mindfulness training (Benn *et al.* 2012).

Mindfulness for carers of ill or elderly

- Caregivers of frail individuals on a mindfulness programme reported reduced depression, stress and burden after the eight-week programme, with further decreases one month later for burden and stress. Calmness and mindful attention also increased (Epstein-Lubow *et al.* 2011).

- A mindfulness programme for families or other carers of elderly nursing home residents reported decreased stress and more satisfaction in their caring role, as well as being able to enjoy time with the person they care for to a greater degree (McBee 2003).

- Family members caring for a parent with dementia found mindfulness training to be more effective at improving their overall mental health, reducing their stress and decreasing their depression than education support (Whitebird *et al.* 2013).

- Mindfulness training and educational interventions decreased stress in family caregivers of dementia relatives (Paller *et al.* 2014).

- Family caregivers of dementia relatives showed significant reductions in depression and anxiety and improvements in perceived self-efficacy after a yoga and meditation intervention. They also reported subjective improvements in physical and emotional functioning (Waelde, Thompson and Gallagher-Thompson 2004).

Mindfulness for carers of people with disabilities

- Adults with profound multiple disabilities presented increased levels of happiness when they were cared for by carers who had undertaken mindfulness training, compared to carers who did not participate in the training (Singh *et al.* 2007).

- Mindfulness training considerably increased the skill of carers to handle the aggressive behaviours individuals with developmental disabilities displayed (Singh *et al.* 2004) and it increased learning and reduced aggression in adults with developmental disability (Singh *et al.* 2006b).

Mindfulness meditation changes the structure of the brain: train your brain to be a better brain.

Evidence for other areas where mindfulness has been found to be helpful

Due to the demanding nature of the work associated with caring, carers may be more likely to experience mental or physical health problems as well as problems in relationships, or even develop an addiction. Here are some further issues with which mindfulness can help.

Relationships

- Mindfulness can improve relationship satisfaction between couples (Carson *et al.* 2006) and help with sexual dysfunction (Blake 2010). It has also been shown to bring about less reactivity and more freedom within relationships and a better understanding of unity, separation, intimacy and independence (Pruitt and McCollum 2010).

- Greater levels of mindfulness are associated with secure attachments (Cordon and Finney 2008).

Addiction

- Mindfulness can assist in stopping addiction relapses (Parks, Anderson and Marlatt 2001) and in retraining the brain in substance misuse (Witkiewitz and Bowen 2010).

- Mindfulness helps with addictive behaviours (Bowen, Chawla and Marlatt 2011).

Mental health

- Mindfulness decreases the secretion of cortisol, a stress hormone (Bowen *et al.* 2011) and stress (Chiesa and Serretti 2009).

- Mindfulness reduces depression and irritation (Baer *et al.* 2006).

- Mindfulness betters our mood and assists in balanced mood overall (Davidson *et al.* 2003).

- Mindfulness and the development of compassion have been found to be inter-related (Tirch 2010).

- Mindfulness assists us in ruminating less and stops relapses of depression (Deyo *et al.* 2009).

- Mindfulness training reduces mind wandering and improves working memory (Mrazek *et al.* 2013).

- Mindfulness reduces anxiety, pain and depression in older people (Smith 2004).

Medical conditions

- Mindfulness assists people with food management (Smith *et al.* 2006).

- Mindfulness reduces sleep interruptions (Winbush, Gross and Kreitzer 2007).

- Mindfulness helps with pain management (Merkes 2010; Garland *et al.* 2012).

- Mindfulness improves immune function (Cresswell *et al.* 2009).

- Mindfulness helps with rheumatoid arthritis, multiple sclerosis, premenstrual syndrome and Type 2 diabetes (Winbush *et al.* 2007).

- Mindfulness lowers blood pressure and reduces chronic migraines (Oberg, Rempe and Bradley 2013).

- Mindfulness brings improvements in quality of life, stress levels and sleep quality in cancer patients (Carlson *et al.* 2003).

- Mindfulness helps with symptoms of fibromyalgia (Grossman *et al.* 2007; Sephton *et al.* 2007; Schmidt *et al.* 2011).

- Mindfulness helps with symptoms of IBS (Garland *et al.* 2012).

- Mindfulness assists with quality of life and fatigue in multiple sclerosis (Grossman *et al.* 2007).

General

- In healthy people, a mindfulness programme reduced stress, anxiety and increased spirituality, values, empathy and self-compassion (Chiesa and Serretti 2009).

- Mindfulness training increases focus (Jha, Krompinger and Baime 2007), decision-making (Haffenbrack, Kinias and Barsado 2013) and working memory (Mrazek *et al.* 2013; Jha *et al.* 2007).

- Mindfulness increases compassion (Tirch 2010).

- Mindfulness helps to increase attention and the regulation of emotions (Tang *et al.* 2007).

Mindfulness practice: Mindful shower

- When you are in the shower or bath, become aware of the water hitting your skin, the warmth of it relaxing your muscles and how it invigorates you. Open your mouth, letting the drops hit your tongue and feeling the water running over your lips and chin.

SUMMARY

- Research has shown mindfulness to be useful and effective for various carer groups.
- Mindfulness is proven to improve people's physical and mental health.

CHAPTER 4

No Quick Fix or Magic Wand

Mindfulness is not a quick fix or magic wand. Early 'ah-ha' moments can provide motivation to continue and benefits can be seen even after a short period of time. However, an ongoing, regular, commitment ensures long-term benefits.

Picture an unmade jigsaw puzzle and imagine it to be your mind with each piece containing different thoughts, emotions and sensations. Without being patient and allowing yourself the time to focus your attention on connecting the pieces, you can never see the whole picture and it will remain scattered.

It is only when you concentrate your attention that all the pieces can gradually be put together and you can become fully aware of what's in front of you. The pieces of your mind that were previously scattered can become connected, making it easier for you to step back and see the bigger picture for what it really is.

Mindfulness practice: Adjusting posture

Take a moment to consider your posture as you read this book. When our mood feels low we often slump in chairs, move more slowly, look down and hunch over. Emotional pain can affect our posture as well as physical pain, leading us to adopt unhealthy positions. On the other hand, when we are confident and calm our shoulders are back, we stand upright, look straight ahead and walk purposefully or sit upright in a chair.

Research has shown that not only do our emotions affect our posture, but our posture can affect our emotions. By adjusting our posture we can lift our mood, reduce aches and pains, improve blood flow around the body and increase our energy levels.

- Sit in a chair in a slumped position for two minutes. Become aware of your breathing and any other sensations. Can you feel any aches? What emotions are present?

- Now sit up straight with your shoulders back. Try to relax your facial muscles and nurture a feeling of calm.

- As you focus on your breathing, notice any changes that occur physically or emotionally. Do you feel more alert or less anxious? If no changes occur, that too is fine.

SUMMARY

- Mindfulness is not a quick fix; you need to do the practices on a regular basis, even if only the short ones.

- Committing to it will ensure long-term benefits as it impacts on the structure of the brain so the more you do it the better the effects.

Part 2

CARER PAINS AND STRAINS

CHAPTER 5

Carers:
The Forgotten Ones

Mindfulness can help you be aware of what you do and the impact it has on your life. Caregivers are a growing group in society yet widely remain an underestimated and undervalued set of people.

- A study found that close to six million people provide informal care in the UK (Office of National Statistics 2011). This included over 100,000 children aged 5–15 acting as carers and over a million adults aged 65 and over.

- In total, only 56 per cent of informal carers (usually caring for relatives) were in good health, compared to people who were not carers, of which 70 per cent were in good health (Doran, Drever and Whitehead 2003).

- The greatest rise has been among those providing over 20 hours care – the point at which caring starts to significantly impact on the health and wellbeing of the carer, and their ability to hold down paid employment alongside their caring responsibilities (Office of National Statistics 2011).

- By 2037, it's anticipated that the number of carers will increase to nine million. Every day another 6000 people take on a caring responsibility – that equals over two million people each year. Over one million people care for more than one person (Office of National Statistics 2011).

- Carers save the UK economy £119 billion per year, an average of £18,473 per carer (Office of National Statistics 2011).

- Over three million people juggle care with work; however the significant demands of caring mean that one in five carers are forced to give up work altogether.

- People providing high levels of care are twice as likely to be permanently sick or disabled. A total of 625,000 people suffer mental and physical ill health as a direct consequence of the stress and physical demands of caring (Office of National Statistics 2011).

The situation in the US is similar (Family Caregiver Alliance 2012; Centers for Disease Control and Prevention 2014):

- A total of 65.7 million caregivers make up 29 per cent of the US adult population providing care to someone who is ill, disabled or aged.

- The majority (83%) are family caregivers – unpaid persons such as family members, friends, and neighbours of all ages who are providing care for a relative or friend.

- About 52 million caregivers provide care to adults (aged 18+) with a disability or illness.

- About 43.5 million adult family caregivers care for someone 50+ years of age and 14.9 million care for someone who has Alzheimer's disease or other dementia.

- Lesbian, gay, bisexual and transgender (LGBT) respondents are slightly more likely to have provided care to an adult friend or relative in the past six months than non-LGBT respondents: 21 per cent vs. 17 per cent.

- Caregiver services were valued at $450 billion per year in 2009 – up from $375 billion in year 2007.

- The value of unpaid family caregivers will likely continue to be the largest source of long-term care services in the US, and the aging population 65+ will more than double between the years 2000 and 2030, increasing to 71.5 million from 35.1 million in 2000.

- Caregivers report having difficulty finding time for themselves (35%), managing emotional and physical stress (29%), and balancing work and family responsibilities (29%).

- Caregivers said they do not go to the doctor because they put their family's needs first (67% said that is a major reason), or they put the care recipient's needs over their own (57%). More than half (51%) said they do not have time to take care of themselves and almost half (49%) said they are too tired to do so.

Developing awareness of ourselves as carers

Many people don't actually identify themselves as carers. This is particularly true if someone, for example, cares for a person part-time or has a child with a chronic condition. They rarely identify themselves and seek support, so it is more difficult for professionals to identify them too. This can lead to carers having more demands than necessary, which can cause physical and mental health issues. Mindfulness can, over time, develop their awareness and their identity of themselves as a caregiver.

Mindfulness practice: A moment of calm in less than two minutes

This breathing practice is an excellent introduction to how focusing on your breathing can help to calm you. It is particularly useful when you feel stressed and it can be performed at any time or in any place when you feel distressed or exhausted. You can even use it to rebalance yourself before or after leaving the person for whom you care.

- Sit in a chair with your eyes open or closed and place one hand on your stomach, feeling the rise and fall of your abdomen. Without forcing your breath in any way, silently count 'in, 2, 3, 4' on the in-breath and 'out, 2, 3, 4' on the out-breath. Repeat this three times.

- Breathe in for the same amount of time as above, but count only 'in, 2, 3' on the in-breath and 'out, 2, 3' on the out-breath. Repeat three times then reduce it to 'in, 2, out, 2' and repeat three times. Now take a breath in and let it out without counting. If this feels difficult say 'in' and then 'out' to the rhythm of your breathing.

- Be aware of how you feel right now. Take this moment of calm with you, knowing that returning to a more balanced state of mind can be as simple as breathing.

SUMMARY

- Acknowledging and accepting the need for support is a sign of strength not weakness.

- Six million people provide informal care in the UK and 65.7 million in the US with caregivers from both countries acknowledging poor health due to the demands of the caring role.

- Actually identifying yourself as a carer is a crucial step in accessing support.

CHAPTER 6

Common Carer Problems

These are some of the common issues that caregivers may experience:

- back, hip or knee problems; shoulder or arm problems; financial struggles; difficulties with balancing employment and caring; maintaining a social life; isolation; lack of time for oneself; lack of care support from family, friends or the wider community; poorer quality of life.

Some signs you could be in distress as a result of your work as a caregiver are:

- mental health: depression and/or anxiety; fearful of the present or the future; anger or frustration; bitterness towards others; high levels of stress; shame or embarrassment; guilt; loneliness; low self-esteem; feeling helpless; more distanced in personal relationships; thoughts of self-harm; loss of interest in previously enjoyed hobbies; social withdrawal.

- physical health: disturbed sleep or insomnia; headaches or migraines; decreased interest in sex; sexual dysfunction; lowered interest in exercise; low levels of energy; fatigue or exhaustion; poor posture; weaker immune response to colds and flu; slower wound healing; increased blood pressure; breathing difficulties; decreased hygiene.

It is also possible that in order to distract yourself from the stresses and worries in your life you focus your attention elsewhere, such as:

- increased risk-taking and impulsive actions; increased use of alcohol or drugs; use of medications such as painkillers; increased or decreased food intake. This may be harmful to you.

Additional emotional problems can arise when the person you care for is a loved one, which is common. If they haven't always been in their current state and were once independent, there can be feelings of loss.

There may also be feelings of guilt thinking you are not caring for the person as well as you should or that you may occasionally be annoyed with them. It can be easy to blame yourself as a carer, but feeling as you do does not mean that you are failing in your task.

🔊 Mindfulness practice: Body Focus

Body Focus practice (use the audio track) focuses your awareness and attention on your body, encouraging you to engage with each area. This practice is particularly good for fatigue or pain.

- Find a quiet place and choose a position which works well for you. Ideally, lie flat on your back on a blanket or carpet, with a cushion for your head if this feels better, or on your bed or sofa.

- Place your legs on a chair, straight or bent, if it is more comfortable when on the floor.

- Cover yourself with a blanket or with something warm as you may become cold.

- If lying down is difficult for you, sit in a chair which provides sufficient support.

- If sitting is not ideal, you can stand steadily against a wall but ensure that you have a chair you can hold onto or sit on should you start to feel unsteady.

- When the audio track says 'breathe into your toes' or any other part of your body, it is metaphorical. Physically we can only breathe into our lungs, so it is about imagining the breath moving through your body, bringing attention to it and relaxing the area.

- If you tend to fall asleep when doing this practice lying down then it is best to do it sitting up.

Once you are familiar with the practice you can try it lying down.

- Listen to the Body Focus practice audio track. After the practice, take a few moments to think about your response to it and if you felt any different afterwards from before. Did you give yourself the time and space to do the practice?

SUMMARY

- Caregivers may struggle and need help physically, mentally, emotionally, socially or financially.
- Mindfulness can assist with identifying symptoms of distress due to your carer role.

CHAPTER 7

The Stress Response

What is the stress response?

The mind and body work together as one unit, not separately. Stress is a complex and difficult experience that we all encounter in our lives, perhaps even daily. By developing your understanding of what exactly stress is and how it impacts on you, you can then use mindfulness to help you reduce the stress response on both your mind and your body.

We often aren't consciously aware of stress on an hourly or daily basis, but research shows that our bodies are continually reacting and interacting with our thoughts and emotions. We tend to see stress as a physical response and don't realise that it starts in our heads before triggering a chain reaction in our bodies.

Evolutionarily, we are built for survival because inherent in our make-up is the profoundly powerful instinct to survive. This instinct is activated in times of threat and, certainly for our ancestors living in a more dangerous and precarious environment, this meant the difference between life and death. A noise behind a bush

may well have held the possibility that a lion was going
to pounce on you and have you for lunch. What then
happens is that your mind's alarm bell is triggered which
activates bodily responses so that you have the power
and energy to fight the lion or to run. However, if the
alarm bell is triggered when there is no real threat but
through demands and tiredness, your mind continues to
perceive this as a real danger so your body continues to
be activated for the flight or fight response.

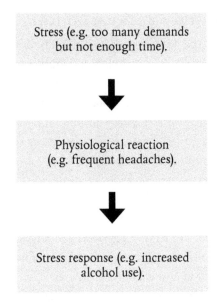

Figure 7.1 How the mind and body interact under stress

In other words, when you experience stress, your mind doesn't realise that you aren't necessarily in real danger and so it reacts as though you may be, or are, confronted with a real threat to your safety. So, even though it is unlikely that there is a lion around the corner as you walk along the road, all those anxious, demanding or stressful thoughts that swirl around your head can be perceived by your mind as danger which then triggers off the stress response and puts you into a state of high alert, even though there is no real danger or lion waiting to pounce. Your mind cannot distinguish between the two situations (perceived danger and actual/real danger) so your body is constantly being activated and over-activated, which is why stress is so damaging. There is also a third type of response, which is the freeze mode, and this is when you stand still or are inactive in the face of stress as a way of protecting yourself.

When you have dealt with the stressor, your body should return to normal over a period of time. A physiological reaction to stress is activated by the sympathetic nervous system putting us into 'go' mode and the process of the body returning to a balanced state is brought about by the parasympathetic system; a 'stop' mode which puts the brakes on. The table below shows what happens to your body during the 'go' and 'stop' modes.

Table 7.1 'Go' and 'Stop' modes	
Sympathetic system – 'go'	Parasympathetic system – 'stop'
Adrenalin and cortisol release.	Noradrenalin released.
Breathing increases.	Breathing slows.
Heart rate increases.	Heart rate decreases.
Energy directed to heart, muscles and the lungs. Digestion decreases/shuts down.	Energy redirected back to the organs that aid in digestion, absorption, excretion and other essential functions.
Feel alert, geared up and ready to go.	Low mood may be felt.

However, when a stressor is continuous, our sympathetic nervous system stays in a repeatedly overactive state. Over a certain period of time this can wear you down which can be a cause of both physical and psychological problems.

The effects of ongoing stress

Stress is implicated in many conditions, meaning that there is a link between stress and the condition, such as:

- organ and memory cells damaged
- distorted thinking
- fatty deposits around waist
- irritable bowel syndrome/stomach problems

- aging

- depression

- hypertension

- rheumatoid arthritis

- diabetes

- cancer

- pain conditions

- sleep disturbance

- infertility, hormonal imbalances, impotence

- loss of libido

- relationship difficulties

- decrease in work performance

- decrease in quality of life

- increase in the use of substances e.g. alcohol or drugs

- increase in risk-taking e.g. gambling or spending money you don't have.

In time, you can become so used to experiencing certain stresses as a carer that they become engrained within you. As little as fleetingly thinking of the person you care for can bring to mind a whole set of concerns with which you've become so familiar. For example, they may be the first thing that pops into your mind when you wake up and you may immediately start to worry, ruminate or make a mental list of all that needs to be done. What if they refuse to let me help them wash again? What if they don't want to eat their breakfast? From thoughts like this you may already feel tired despite having just woken.

When you woke you didn't consciously decide you would feel like this. It was as if by magic these thoughts popped into your mind and began to take on a life of their own, even in your half-awake state. Using the mindfulness practices regularly can help you become aware of what you're feeling and how to manage these feelings in a different way. It could mean that the next time you find yourself in that situation, you can acknowledge, 'I'm stressing about this.' Having a moment to yourself when you wake can help you gain more perspective on how you feel and how you react to it. One suggestion is to sit on the side of your bed and take a few breaths to focus yourself before rushing off to start your day.

Remember, it is your day regardless of all the demands on your time and energy.

Mindfulness practice: Mindful eating

This practice can be done on your own or with the person for whom you care. It can bring more calm to meal times and allow both parties to enjoy the flavours of their food and increase the experience of eating.

- Take a piece of fruit, chocolate or any food that is not too difficult to chew. Eat it as normal. Now take another piece, place it on your tongue and let it sit there.

- Without chewing, focus on the sensation. What does it feel like? Can you identify a taste that you had not noticed on the previous piece? Chew the food slowly. Does the chewing make a sound? Is it difficult to resist the urge to swallow the food?

Mindfulness allows you to step back from your feelings, thoughts and actions which, in turn, lets you choose how you wish to respond to them.

SUMMARY

- The stress response is necessary for our survival but it can have negative effects on the mind and body when it is activated too often, which carers are vulnerable to.

- Mindfulness can help in reducing the activation of the stress response which can then help to reduce the symptoms of stress and their damaging effects.

CHAPTER 8

Seeing Yourself as a Whole

What is the biopsychosocial model?

This model highlights the distinct features influencing a person's wellbeing and shows that the way we are is directed by our biology, our psychology and the social environment that surrounding us.

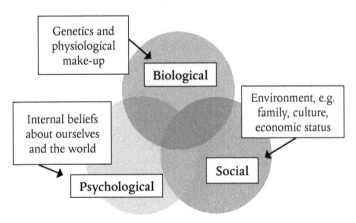

Figure 8.1 The biopsychosocial model

How can the biopsychosocial model be applied to caregivers?

The biopsychosocial model can aid our understanding of the relationship between the mind and the body and how they interact. All three factors – biological, psychological and social are equally important in defining who we are as people in the present and how we go about our carer roles.

Many of our physical and some psychological attributes are inherited from our parents through our genes; however it is our experiences growing up which shape our development.

Take for example the process of growing a flower in a pot. All of the plant's biological make-up is contained within the seed, but its growth and characteristics will also be affected by how often you water it, how much sunlight it receives, the nutrients in the soil and other environmental factors. Similarly, humans inherit traits from their parents but their experiences, particularly in early development, lay the foundation for their psychological and emotional make-up which will have an influence throughout their lives (Rezek 2010).

What is the psychodynamic approach?

Central to the 'psycho' part of the biopsychosocial model is the psychodynamic approach. The psychodynamic approach is founded on the concept that our early experiences have a significant impact, often unconsciously, on how we are in adulthood. The general theory is that if we are provided with consistent love and affection in our early years, then as adults we will think of ourselves as lovable and valuable. However, if our care in early years is inconsistent, lacking, or even abusive then this can impact negatively on how we see ourselves and behave in adulthood (Rezek 2010).

A child's view of themselves and the world is developed throughout these early years. Their education in what is good and bad and whether they are behaving well or not comes in this period of early life too, as well as learning whether they are worthy and competent (Rezek 2010).

How can the psychodynamic approach be applied to carers?

We bring into our adult lives the experiences we had as children. Therefore, the relationships we had with our parents can influence how we are as a carer and how we develop relationships with the people for whom we now care.

- An example: an individual's father may have been short-tempered with them as a child and gone from one extreme to another. One hour he would be loving, the next he would be irritable. This could unconsciously influence the individual in their own care work as an adult, such as easily losing their temper or feeling extremes of emotions more frequently. Alternatively, another individual's parents could have given them a consistently loving upbringing, helping them to be able to form stable, balanced relationships and to be patient and tolerant adults, qualities that will help them as carers. However, this is not to say that people who had difficult childhoods aren't loving adult carers. It is only highlighting how patterns can so easily be repeated.

- On the opposite side, if a child had parents who implied that nothing was good enough or enough, then that child could easily become a caregiver who finds it difficult to set boundaries and who runs the risk of giving so much of themselves that they become physically unwell or depressed.

Summary

In terms of any distress you may currently feel as a caregiver, it is not necessarily true that one factor will be the cause of another. However, biological, psychological, social and early life experiences are inevitably interlinked. By being aware of these factors, you can find out more about how you developed to be the person you are today and what makes you do the things you do. Mindfulness can be of value here too as it can allow you to gain greater perspective on your life. Think of some of the different factors that may have contributed to who you are, what you presently think and feel, and how you respond to different situations.

Biological	Psychological	Social	Early life experiences

By knowing your past influences, you give
yourself a chance to better understand
how they impact on your present life.

IMPORTANT

By starting to engage more with yourself as a whole and by understanding the events that have brought you to where you are now, feelings and memories may be brought into view which could be upsetting. Should this happen, acknowledge them but manage them by listening to music or talking to a friend, for example. If the feelings are too distressing, you should speak to a qualified therapist. Therapy should not be regarded as intimidating; it is simply two people coming together to take care of your life and develop your understanding of your feelings so that you can manage them in a helpful way.

SUMMARY

- We may think about our minds and bodies as separate entities, but they constantly interact with, and influence, each other.

- Biological, psychological and social factors, including childhood experiences, influence our personalities and shape who we are and the way we see the world.

Part 3

HOW CAN I BREAK
THE CHAIN?

CHAPTER 9

Living in the Present

Have you ever found yourself in a situation as a caregiver that you would have preferred to avoid? Perhaps you can't seem to shake the feeling that you don't do enough for the person for whom you care or you shouted then regretted it? An approach that can help is learning how to be more aware of your responses in the present moment.

By centring your attention on this moment in time, it gives you awareness and insight into what is happening right now and how you respond to it. Your wellbeing is often influenced by thinking about past experiences so by shifting to the now, this moment, you can start to recognise what you are doing and choose how to respond differently rather than automatically repeat the cycle of thoughts, feelings or behaviours.

The purpose of mindfulness is not to erase
or avoid thoughts, sensations and emotions.
The aim is to become more aware of them
and let them be rather than fight them.

◀)) Mindfulness practice: The Mountain meditation

The Mountain meditation is designed to create a sense of stability, balance and wellbeing. It is about claiming this moment and this space for yourself and anchoring yourself no matter how distressing life may be. It is a reminder of your inner resilience, reassuring you that you can weather the storms in life.

- When doing this practice, ensure that you stand on a non-slip surface and have a chair you can hold onto if you are unsteady on your feet. Alternatively, you can do this practice sitting in a chair if necessary.

- Listen to The Mountain meditation audio track.

- Afterwards, take a few moments to reflect on how you face difficulties. Think about the storms you have weathered, the times when you thought that you could not cope or that life was not going to get any better. Hold in your mind what you think helped you to get through them.

No matter how chaotic life may seem at times, you have the ability to develop resilience. Even when you feel you are struggling, you often find a strength within yourself that you can draw on to help you manage the pain, fear, distress and despair that life can inflict.

Thoughts, emotions and experiences are transient, but the core of you is constant and enduring. By engaging in practices such as The Mountain, you are reinforcing your capacity to choose wellbeing over distress.

Mindfulness is as much about celebrating your achievements, success, health and wellbeing as it is about negotiating the more difficult experiences of your life.

SUMMARY

- Learning how to live in the present can help you break the cycles you get caught in.
- Centring your attention on the present aids your awareness of what you are truly thinking and feeling in the here and now.

CHAPTER 10

A Reactive Mind: Stop and Choose

It can sometimes be demanding and difficult staying calm whilst caring for a person. For example, you may care for someone who repeatedly displays challenging behaviours in spite of your efforts. At moments like these, patience can wear thin and frustration or despair can mount. Mindfulness practices can help you to develop the ability to step back and think about how you want to act, rather than react.

STOP...BREATHE...ACT

When you actively avoid the thoughts that make you feel distressed, it can make them more intense in the long-term (Hayes and Feldman 2004). While thoughts are part of what makes you who you are, they don't exist outside of your mind. By using the practices, when you notice yourself having distressing thoughts you will be able to make the choice as to how you act upon them.

Thoughts are not facts; they are transitory
statements or questions that come and go,
shift and change. You are not defined by
your thoughts so you don't need to attach
to them. They are only thoughts so you
can choose how you wish to use them.

To encourage yourself to stop and
consider before making decisions is a
way of taking charge of your life.

Decisions, decisions...

Bring to mind a distressing situation as a caregiver that
you sometimes experience. For example, the person you
care for is relentlessly demanding of your attention,
which you find exhausting and frustrating. Perhaps
you feel upset and want to cry or you may want a glass
of wine. View the decision you make as you would a
multiple choice question in an exam. You don't have
only one option in front of you but several. If you stop
and be mindful of the option you choose, you may then
feel as if you have more control over the situation. So, for
example, instead of getting a glass of wine you go for a
walk or do two minutes of breathing. On the following
page is a table for you to keep track of how mindfulness
is helping you learn a more considered approach to
making decisions.

Situations where I tend to react negatively	How I now respond to the situations using mindfulness

Mindfulness practice: Choosing to refocus

- If you notice any distressing thoughts, take a few mindful breaths, anchoring yourself to the present while you observe the thought. Recognise that it is only a thought and that you do not need to attach any significance to it.

- Sit quietly with any emotions associated with the thought, then start to shift your attention onto an aspect of your present experience that feels kinder; perhaps the warmth of the sunshine or the soft rug under your feet. No matter how small, appreciate it.

- Choosing to refocus your attention is a step towards developing emotional resilience.

SUMMARY

- Mindfulness practices can allow us to develop space and time to think and act, not react.

- We can learn that we have a choice when it comes to how we act on our thoughts.

CHAPTER 11

Management of Distress

Feelings of 'how did this happen' or 'why', even 'why me?' can often arise when times are hard and it can be difficult to manage distressing experiences. Through your developed awareness gained from doing the mindfulness practices, you can become more attuned to your distress and, in turn, become more accepting of it. Everyone experiences suffering at some point as it is part of our human existence. It isn't the only experience we go through, but how we respond to these experiences can influence our happiness.

Research has illustrated that Buddhist caregivers of seriously mentally ill relatives in Thailand judged that suffering and acceptance were major elements of their perspective on what caregiving requires (Hayes and Feldman 2004). Research has also discovered that mindfulness practices based around the themes of acceptance can be of particular use for older people, as deteriorating biological systems, chronic disease, being cared for and suffering are inevitable parts of later life (Sethabouppha and Kane 2005).

Sometimes we can feel so distressed by our suffering that we become frightened of it or even angry about it, so we push it into the depths of our minds rather than face the power of it. Once we bring it into clear view, which mindfulness helps with, we can begin to observe and accept it rather than trying to ignore or fight it all the time. Mindfulness can help you hold onto the good times you have and help you to strive towards a better quality of life in a considered, balanced way.

 ## Mindfulness practice: Mindful Awareness

Mindful Awareness is about becoming aware of what is happening within yourself and working with it. On the MP3 audio track download, there are two Mindful Awareness breathing practices, one of five minutes in length and another that is 20 minutes. Begin with the five-minute version (Mindful Breathing) and then move on to the 20-minute version (Mindful Awareness). There is also a track entitled Gentle Space which is five minutes of silence interspersed with 'bong' sounds. This can be used if you wish to sit silently for five minutes but find your mind wandering. The 'bong' sounds remind you to come back to focusing on your breathing. Ideally, do the 20-minute version a few times per week and the five-minute one on the other days.

- This practice is not about emptying your mind of all thoughts but more about finding an anchor of balance and calm within yourself.

- Positions: as with the Body Focus practice, you can lie on the floor, sit or stand when doing this practice, but it is best to try sitting in a chair in an upright but relaxed and open manner.

- Find a time and place where you won't be interrupted and know that you can remain focused on the meditation even if there is noise around you.

- Listen to the Mindful Awareness practice of your choice.

Tracking your progress

It is helpful to take a moment to reflect on your progress. Perhaps a week or two after practising mindful awareness go over your experience so far. Have you noticed any effects of the practices? Have you been managing stressful situations differently?

Think about your attitudes towards the practices. Have you given yourself the time to focus on them or have you put them off? Your attitude towards these practices can reveal aspects of your approach towards other areas of your life.

If you have been hesitant about starting then perhaps this stage will be a turning point for your motivation.

With each breath is a new beginning. If you have approached the practices in a motivated manner, take a moment to think about what has brought you this far. Holding on to this motivation can help to develop your own sense of resilience and belief that you can make a difference in your life.

Letting go of control can give us more control.

SUMMARY

- Mindful awareness enables you to become more attuned to your distressing experiences.
- Reflecting on your experiences of suffering in a kind and gentle way can help to increase your acceptance of them and give you a way of taking care of, and managing, them.

CHAPTER 12

Self-care

We tend not to pause and feel kindness towards ourselves for all that we do. This can be particularly true of carers. A self-care practice creates a feeling of compassion towards yourself and others. In addition, when you are feeling distressed it can help you to be less critical of yourself and kinder towards yourself.

Mindfulness practice: Self-care practice

This meditation is a starting point for developing a kind and caring attitude towards yourself. Sit quietly in any position that is comfortable for you and take a few breaths to settle. Repeat the following phrases to yourself:

- May I be happy and healthy.
- May I accept myself for all that I am.
- May I live my life with ease.

Repeat these phrases a number of times even when it feels difficult, as when we are distressed we can start to doubt that we are worthy and deserving of happiness. You can change the wording to suit your own ideas of generosity, kindness and care towards yourself.

You may find your attention begins to wander and this is to be expected as that is what minds do. Gently bring your attention back to the practice. Each time your mind wanders and you bring it back to your breathing you're encouraging your physical brain to make positive connections and your emotional mind to pay attention to the good.

Mindfulness practice: Making time to care for yourself

A danger when you're a caregiver is that your life becomes focused on someone else's needs to the exclusion of yours. If you continually deny your own needs then you run the risk of burnout and ill-health. What is often difficult for carers to take on board is that they need to be as responsible for their own psychological and physical health as much as for the person for whom they are caring.

The expected response is, 'I know that but I don't have time.' There may well be very limited time for yourself so it is particularly important that you make good use of the time you do have. Some of the practices can be done within minutes or seconds and can quickly lead to a psychological and physical change within you. The difficult part is getting yourself to the point of recognising that you are allowed to put aside time to care for yourself. This is essential if you are to take care of your own life.

There will often be a nagging thought in your head trying to persuade you that you don't have enough time, or that makes you feel guilty for taking a break. Acknowledge these thoughts but put them aside and ensure you do something for yourself each week, no matter how small.

SUMMARY

- We can be very harsh on ourselves despite all the good that we do as carers.
- Self-care practices create a sense of kindness and compassion towards ourselves and others.

Part 4

STAYING COMMITTED
BRINGS LONG-TERM GAINS

CHAPTER 13

Setting Boundaries

In order to take care of your own life it is important that you set boundaries. If your demands leave you stretched for time, give yourself the best possible chance to make time for yourself so that you have the opportunity to develop your mindfulness practice.

Setting boundaries around your workload

Modern society seems to mean being busy. Technology and social media have resulted in many people rarely having time for themselves (Rezek 2012). So often when you ask people how they are, the response is, 'I'm ok… busy,' as though busy is somehow an indicator that life is fulfilling. Many of you have the demands of careers, families and taking care of yourself and caring is an additional workload you need to manage. Sometimes being busy can help you to avoid difficult feelings, which is not always helpful.

Mindfulness practice:
Releasing the grip

- Take a moment to focus on something in your life that is a source of suffering. It may be a demand of some sort as a carer. Perhaps you've not had the opportunity to fully acknowledge what it is and where it has come from. It may feel like a knot in your mind or as if it is a hand that is tightly clenched, unwilling to open. Over a period of time, we can lock our despair into a dark place in our minds where it can't be found and therefore can't be taken care of in a helpful way.

- Focus on all the distress it causes you, whether it be mental or physical. Does it really deserve to take so much out of you? Try to soften your view of it. Let it be and if possible, see it with kindness.

- Allow the grip to slowly open, releasing the tension it holds by breathing into the image, letting it ease with each breath. You can use whatever imagery works for you when you are feeling distress. It can be an additional aid in extending your awareness of yourself and the things that leave you feeling tense and worried.

Doing the practices shouldn't be seen as a chore. It is a time for you and only you. For example, after a long day at work or having carried out a difficult task, it can be used to release tension and to rebalance yourself. There is no right or wrong way with mindfulness, but the more you do it the more it helps psychologically and physiologically. Use whichever practices you like on a regular basis. If you think it will help, try explaining to your family, friends or partner the basics of mindfulness and why you're practising it. They too might want to try it as they could benefit from it as will the people around them.

SUMMARY

- Boundaries are an important and necessary form of protection and self-care. They need to be put in place and respected if you are to take care of your own wellbeing.

- Mindfulness practices aren't a chore or item on a list but a time to renew and rebalance.

CHAPTER 14

Resistance

Stick with it

Resistance to doing the practices can happen at any time. It may be happening already by not finding time for the practices or perhaps your mind may resist doing the rest of the practice and wander elsewhere when you are partway through it. Every time you refocus your concentration back to the practice, your mind becomes stronger psychologically and in terms of your brain connections, and this is one way of developing resilience.

Another challenge you may find is staying with a difficult thought that comes to mind during a practice. Pushing away difficult thoughts and feelings as a coping strategy is commonly used, but is not always helpful. Acknowledge these thoughts rather than push them away. Observe what comes up and then let it be there without delving into or reacting to it and then let it pass on. Letting it pass on is different from the idea of not worrying about it or even dismissing it. Letting it pass on is like seeing it as a cloud that drifts and changes shape as it moves across the sky.

You may be tempted to put this programme aside and not use it or to stop at a later stage. There may be some practices you feel aren't as useful or some concepts you disagree with. That is fine; mindfulness is about finding what works best for you. Expecting mindfulness to fix your life is not realistic. However, with time it can assist you to become more able to face your thoughts and emotions in a balanced way and to respond to yourself and your life in a way where you have choice. It develops a belief in your own capacity to manage yourself and your life even when it feels awful but it also gives you the awareness to be able to enjoy those good moments too.

There is no end point with mindfulness. Each moment of life is a new one which can be reacted to with fear or responded to with awareness.

SUMMARY

- Do not feel disheartened if resistance occurs, simply refocus.
- Mindfulness is all about finding which practices and concepts work best for you.

CHAPTER 15

The Benefits

As you continue to practise mindfulness, you will begin to reap the benefits in your work as a caregiver as well as in other areas of your life.

> *Mindfulness meditation can change the neuronal pathways in the brain: the more you do it the more your brain responds.*

You may want to track your progress, so below are some questions for you to consider on the benefits that mindfulness is giving you.

- Can you identify one time and place where you are able to practise mindfulness if only for five minutes a day?

- Which mindfulness practices have been most helpful for you and why?

- In which situations would you benefit most by being mindful?

- What is the one thing, above all others, that you have learnt about yourself from practising mindfulness?

Mindfulness should provide you with an ever-growing resource to deal with the demands of being a caregiver. It encourages and trains you to be more aware of yourself in the present moment and to actually be in the present rather than think of the past or future. It creates and develops resilience, stability and a sense of groundedness within you. Ultimately, it should help you take care of yourself while you care for others.

Mindfulness can help with those harsh and difficult thoughts and emotions that carers may carry.

Being mindful will help you to recognise the kindness, generosity, compassion and strength that you have and give to those for whom you care.

SUMMARY

- Tracking your progress is a useful way to gauge the benefits that mindfulness is bringing to your life.

- Mindfulness provides an ever-growing resource to cope with the caregiver role.

No one can take care of you except yourself.

ABOUT THE AUTHOR

Dr Cheryl Rezek is a Consultant Clinical Psychologist who has worked across various fields of mental health for many years. She has combined clinical and academic work, run a doctoral clinical psychology specialist teaching unit, headed services, developed numerous treatment programmes and provided consultation, teaching and supervision to a broad set of professionals and organisations as well as lectured on an extensive range of topics to health professionals, commercial leaders and managers, and to the public. She has worked with children, adolescents and adults in many different areas including learning disabilities, substance misuse, severe mental health, secure psychiatric units and a hospice for terminally ill patients and their families. She developed a model of working that allows for making psychological principles and mindfulness work accessible to a broad audience, from the general public to organisations, leaders and decision-makers, in a straightforward and accessible manner. This model (affectionately known as Life Happens) is based on her extensive clinical experience and it encourages awareness of oneself within a context, the development of resilience and skills and the use of mindfulness. She has a clinical practice, authors work, consults and runs workshops nationally and internationally. She is on the committee for the British Psychological Society's Good Practice Guidelines on Mindfulness and her model is regarded as an emerging mindfulness-based approach.

Visit the author's website:

www.lifehappens-mindfulness.com.

Other work available by the author

Life Happens: Waking up to yourself and your life in a mindful way (2010). Leachcroft.
Book + 2 CDs. Available as a print book with CDs or an EBook via www.lifehappens-mindfulness.com

Brilliant Mindfulness: How the mindful approach can help you towards a better life (2012). Pearson.
Book + CD. Available as a print book and Kindle

iMindfulness on the go
An app with audio and written material to take with you wherever you go. See www.lifehappens-mindfulness.com or your app store

Quit Smoking with Mindfulness and Change Your Life Forever: A pocket guide to help stop smoking and other addictions.
www.lifehappens-mindfulness.com

Mindfulness for Anxiety and Depression: A pocket guide to help you find a way through the struggle
www.lifehappens-mindfulness.com

Mindfulness for the Symptoms of Cancer: A pocket guide to help manage the distress and pain.
www.lifehappens-mindfulness.com

Mindfulness for 8–12 year olds: A gentle and enjoyable way to learn a skill for life.
www.lifehappens-mindfulness.com

Mindfulness Meditations MP3 (Body Focus, three Mindful Awareness/Breathing Meditations, Mindful Movement).
Available as an MP3 download via www.lifehappens-mindfulness.com

REFERENCES

Allen, B., Chambers, R. and Knight, W. (Melbourne Academic Mindfulness Group) (2006). 'Mindfulness-based psychotherapies: A review of conceptual foundations, empirical evidence and practical considerations.' *Australian and New Zealand Journal of Psychiatry 40*, 4, 285–294.

Baer, R.A., Smith, G.T., Hopkins, J., Kreitemeyer, J. and Toney, L. (2006) 'Using self report assessment methods to explore facets of mindfulness.' *Assessment 13*, 1, 27–45.

Baker, S. (2014) *Does mindfulness mediate the influence of stress upon parenting relationships in a foster care population? A pilot study of the effectiveness of a mindfulness-based parenting program for foster carers.* Summary of thesis available at www.findlab.net.au/research-findings/does-mindfulness-mediate-the-influence-of-stress-upon-parenting-relationships-in-a-foster-care-population-a-pilot-study-of-the-effectiveness-of-a-mindfulness-based-parenting-program-for-foster-carers/, accessed 21 February 2015.

Bazarko, D., Cate, R.A., Azocar, F. and Kreitzner, M.J. (2013) 'The impact of an innovative mindfulness-based stress reduction program on the health and well-being of nurses employed in a corporate setting.' *Journal of Workplace Behavioral Health 28*, 2, 107–133.

Benn, R., Akiva, T., Ariel, S. and Roesner, R. (2012) 'Mindfulness training effects for parents and educators of children with special needs.' *Developmental Psychology 48*, 5, 1476–1487.

Blake, C. (2010) *The Joy of Mindful Sex: Be in the Moment and Enrich your Lovemaking.* Lewes: Ivy Press.

Bögels, S.M., Lehtonen, A. and Restifo, K. (2010) 'Mindful parenting in mental health care.' *Mindfulness 1*, 2, 107–120.

Bowen, S., Chawla, N. and Marlatt, A.G. (2011) *Mindfulness-Based Relapse Prevention for Addictive Behaviours: A Clinician's Guide.* New York: Guilford Press.

Carlson, L.E., Speca, M., Patel, K.D. and Goodey, E. (2003) 'Mindfulness-based stress reduction in relation to quality of life, mood, symptoms of stress, and immune parameters in breast and prostate cancer outpatients.' *Psychosomatic Medicine 65*, 571–581.

Carson, J.W., Carson, K.M., Gill, K.M. and Baucom, D.H. (2006) 'Mindfulness Based Relationship Enhancement (MBRE) in Couples.' In R.A. Baer (ed.) *Mindfulness Based Treatment Approaches: Clinician's Guide to Evidence Base and Applications.* Burlington, MA: Elsevier.

Centers for Disease Control and Prevention (2014) Health Aging Program, Atlanta, USA. Family Caregiving Facts. Available at www.cdc.gov/aging/caregiver/facts, accessed 21 February 2015.

Chiesa, A. and Serretti, A. (2009) 'Mindfulness-based stress reduction for stress management in healthy people: A review and meta-analysis.' *Journal of Alternative and Complementary Medicine 15*, 5, 593.

Cordon, S.L. and Finney, S.J. (2008) 'Measurement invariance of the mindful attention awareness scale across adult attachment style.' *Measurement and Evaluation in Counseling and Development 40*, 4, 18.

Cresswell, J.D., Myers, H.F., Cole, S.W. and Irwin, M.R. (2009) 'Mindfulness meditation training effects on CD4+ T lymphocytes in HIV-1 infected adults: A small randomized controlled trial.' *Brain, Behavior and Immunity 23*, 2, 86–97.

Davidson, R.J., Kabat-Zinn, J., Schumacher, M., Rosenkranz, D. *et al.* (2003) 'Alterations in brain and immune function produced by mindfulness meditation.' *Psychosomatic Medicine 65*, 4, 564–570.

Deyo, M., Wilson, K, A., Ong, J. and Koopman, C. (2009) 'Mindfulness and rumination: Does mindfulness training lead to reductions in the ruminative thinking associated with depression?' EXPLORE: *Journal of Science and Healing 5*, 5, 265–271.

Doran, T., Drever, F. and Whitehead, M. (2003) 'Health of young and elderly informal carers: analysis of UK census data.' *BMJ (Clinical Research Edition) 327*, 7428, 1388.

Epstein-Lubow, G., McBee, L., Darling, E., Armey, M. and Miller, I.W. (2011) 'A pilot investigation of mindfulness-based stress reduction for caregivers of frail elderly.' *Mindfulness 2*, 2, 95–102.

Family Caregiver Alliance (2012) National Center on Caregiving Selected Caregiver Statistics, available at www.caregiver.org/selected-caregiver-statistics, accessed 21 February 2015.

Foueur, M., Besley, K., Burton, G., Yu, N. and Crisp. J. (2013) 'Enhancing the resilience of nurses and midwives: A pilot of a mindfulness-based program for increased health, sense of coherence and decreased depression, anxiety and stress.' *Contemporary Nurse 45*, 1, 114–125.

Fourtney, L., Luchterhand, C., Zakletskaia, L., Zgierska, A. and Rakel, D. (2013) 'Abbreviated mindfulness intervention for job satisfaction, quality of life, and compassion in primary care physicians: A pilot study.' *Annals of Family Medicine 11*, 5, 412–420.

Garland, E.L., Gaylord, S.A., Palsson, O., Faurot, K., Mann, J.D. and Whitehead, W.E. (2012) 'Therapeutic mechanisms of a mindfulness-based treatment for IBS: Effects on visceral sensitivity, catastrophizing, and affective processing of pain sensations.' *Journal of Behavioral Medicine 35*, 6, 591–602.

Goodman, M.J. and Schorling, B. (2012) 'A mindfulness course decreases burnout and improves wellbeing among healthcare providers.' *International Journal of Psychiatry Medicine 43*, 2, 119–128.

Grossman, P., Tiefenthaler-Gilmer, U., Raysz, A. and Kesper, U. (2007) 'Mindfulness training as an intervention for fibromyalgia: evidence of postintervention and 3-year follow-up benefits in well-being.' *Psychotherapy and Psychosomatics 76*, 226–233.

Grossman, P., Kappos, L., Gensicke, H., D'Souza, M., Mohr, D.C., Penner, I. K., *et al.* (2010) 'MS quality of life, depression, and fatigue improve after mindfulness training: a randomized trial.' *Neurology 75*, 1141–1149.

Haffenbrack, A., Kinias, Z. and Barsado, S. (2013) 'Debasing the mind through meditation: Mindfulness and the sunk-cost bias.' *Psychological Science 25*, 2, 369–379.

Hayes, A.M. and Feldman, G. (2004) 'Clarifying the construct of mindfulness in the context of emotion regulation and the process of change in therapy.' *Clinical Psychology: Science and Practice 11*, 3, 255–262.

Jha A.P., Krompinger J. and Baime, M.J. (2007) 'Mindfulness training modifies subsystems of attention.' *Cognitive Affective and Behavioral Neuroscience 7*, 109–119.

MacKenzie, C.S., Poulin, P.A. and Seidman-Carlson, R. (2006) 'A brief mindfulness-based stress reduction intervention for nurses and nurse aides.' *Applied Nursing Research 19*, 2, 105–109.

Martín-Asuero, A. and García-Banda, G. (2010) 'The mindfulness-based stress reduction program (MBSR) reduces stress related psychological distress in healthcare professionals.' *Spanish Journal of Psychology 13*, 2, 897–905.

McBee, L. (2003) 'Mindfulness practice with the frail elderly and their caregivers.' *Topics in Geriatric Rehabilitation 19*, 4, 257–264.

Merkes, M. (2010) 'Mindfulness based stress reduction for people with chronic disease.' *Australian Journal of Primary Health 16*, 3, 200–210.

Minor, H.G., Carlson, L.E., Mackenzie, M.J., Zernicke, K. and Jones, L. (2006) 'Evaluation of a mindfulness-based stress reduction (MBSR) program for caregivers of children with chronic conditions.' *Social Work in Health Care 43*, 1, 91–109.

Mrazek, M.D., Franklin, M.S., Phillips, D.T., Baird, B. and Schooler, J.W. (2013) 'Mindfulness training improves working memory capacity and GRE performance while reducing mind wandering.' *Psychological Science 24*, 5, 776–781.

Oberg, E.B., Rempe, M. and Bradley, R. (2013) 'Self-directed mindfulness training and improvement in blood pressure, migraine frequency, and quality of life.' *Global Advances in Health and Medicine 2*, 2, 20–25.

Office of National Statistics (2011) Available at www.ons.gov.uk/ons/rel/census/2011-census/key-statistics-for-local-authorities-in-england-and-wales/stb-2011-census-key-statistics-for-england-and-wales, accessed 1 January 2015.

Paller K.A., Creery, J.D., Florczak, S.M., Weintraub, S., *et al.* (2014) 'Benefits of mindfulness training for patients with progressive cognitive decline and their caregivers.' *American Journal of Alzheimer's Disease and Other Dementias.* DOI: 10.1177/1533317514545377. Published online. Available at http://aja.sagepub.com, accessed 1 January 2015.

Parks, G.A., Anderson, B.K. and Marlatt, G.A. (2001) *Interpersonal Handbook of Alcohol Dependence and Problems.* New York: John Wiley.

Pruitt, I.T. and McCollum, E.E. (2010) 'Voices of experienced meditators: The impact of meditation practice on intimate relationships.' *Contemporary Family Therapy 32*, 2, 135–154.

Regehr, C., Glancy, D. and Leblanc, V.R. (2014) 'Interventions to reduce the consequences of stress in physicians: A review and meta-analysis.' *Journal of Nervous Mental Disorder 202*, 5, 353–359.

Rezek, C.A. (2010) *Life Happens: Waking up to Yourself and Your Life in a Mindful Way.* London: Leachcroft.

Rezek, C.A. (2012) *Brilliant Mindfulness: How the Mindful Approach Can Help You Towards a Better Life.* Harlow: Pearson.

Rushton, C.H., Kaszniak, A.W. and Halifax, J.S. (2013) 'A framework for understanding moral distress among palliative care clinicians.' *Journal of Palliative Medicine 16*, 1074–1079.

Schmidt, S., Grossman, P., Schwarzer, B., Jena, S., Naumann, J. and Walach, H. (2011) 'Treating fibromyalgia with mindfulness-based stress reduction: results from a 3-armed randomized controlled trial.' *Pain 152*, 361–369.

Sephton, S.E., Salmon, P., Weissbecker, I., Ulmer, C., *et al.* (2007) 'Mindfulness meditation alleviates depressive symptoms in women with fibromyalgia: results of a randomized clinical trial.' *Arthritis and Rheumatism 57*, 77–78.

Sethabouppha, H. and Kane, C. (2005) 'Caring for the seriously mentally ill in Thailand: Buddhist family caregiving.' *Archives of Psychiatric Nursing 19*, 2, 44–57.

Shapiro, S.L., Astin, J.A., Bishop, S.R. and Cordova, M. (2005) 'Mindfulness-based stress reduction for health care professionals: Results from a randomized trial.' *International Journal of Stress Management 12*, 164–176.

Shapiro, S.L., Schwartz, G.E. and Bonner, G. (1998) 'Effects of mindfulness-based stress reduction on medical and premedical students.' *Journal of Behavioral Medicine 21*, 581–599.

Shier, M.L. and Graham, J.R. (2010) 'Mindfulness, subjective well-being, and social work: Insight into their interconnection from social work practitioners.' *Social Work Education 30*, 1, 29–44.

Singh, N.N., Lancioni, G.E., Winton, A.S., Curtis, W.J., Wahler, R.G., Sabaawi, M., *et al.* (2006b) 'Mindful staff increase learning and reduce aggression in adults with developmental disabilities.' *Research in Developmental Disabilities 27*, 5, 545–558.

Singh, N.N., Lancioni, G.E., Winton, A.S., Singh, J., Curtis, W.J., Wahler, R.G., *et al.* (2007) 'Mindful parenting decreases aggression and increases social behavior in children with developmental disabilities.' *Behavior Modification 31*, 6, 749–771.

Singh, N.N., Lancioni, G.E., Winton, A.S., Wahler, R.G., Singh, J. and Sage, M. (2004) 'Mindful caregiving increases happiness among individuals with profound multiple disabilities.' *Research in Developmental Disabilities 25*, 2, 207–218.

Singh, N.N., Singh, S.D., Sabaawi, M., Myers, R.E. and Wahler, R.G. (2006a) 'Enhancing treatment team process through mindfulness-based mentoring in an inpatient psychiatric hospital.' *Behavior Modification 30*, 4, 423–441.

Smith, A. (2004) 'Clinical uses of mindfulness training for older people.' *Behavioural and Cognitive Psychotherapy 32*, 4, 423–430.

Smith, W.B., *et al.* (2006) 'A preliminary study of the effects of a modified mindfulness intervention on binge eating.' *Complementary Health Practice Review 11*, 3, 133–143.

Tang, Y.Y., Ma, Y., Wang, J., Fan, Y. *et al.* (2007) 'Short-term meditation training improves attention and self-regulation.' *Proceedings of the National Academy of Sciences USA 104*, 43, 17152–17156.

Tirch, D.D. (2010) 'Mindfulness as a context for the cultivation of compassion.' *International Journal of Cognitive Therapy 3*, 2, 113–123.

Waelde, L.C. Thompson, L. and Gallagher-Thompson, D. (2004) 'A pilot study of yoga and meditation intervention for dementia caregiver stress.' *Journal of Clinical Psychology 60*, 6, 677–687.

Whitebird, R.R., Kreitzer, M., Crain, A.L., Lewis, B.A., Hanson, L.R. and Enstad, C.J. (2013) 'Mindfulness-based stress reduction for family caregivers: A randomized controlled trial.' *The Gerontologist 5*, 4, 676–686.

Winbush, N.Y., Gross, C.R. and Kreitzer, M.J. (2007) 'The effects of mindfulness based stress reduction on sleep disturbance: A systematic review.' *Explore (NY) 3*, 6, 585–591.

Witkiewitz, K. and Bowen, S. (2010) 'Depression, craving and substance use following a randomized trial of mindfulness-based relapse prevention.' *Journal of Consulting and Clinical Psychology 78*, 3, 362–374.